Ethical Decision Making

for

Helping Professionals

Subtle Boundary Dilemmas

Sheila McGuire, L.S.W., C.C.D.P.

HAZELDEN

About the workbook. This workbook introduces ethical issues surrounding the ways that people establish and maintain boundaries in the helping relationship. With appropriate boundaries, clients can begin their journey to healing. But when boundaries are breached, clients can feel angry, confused, depressed, and suspicious. Boundaries between client and professional are part of this equation; so are boundaries between professionals. This workbook examines both areas.

We recognize that helping professionals must also attend to boundary concerns that arise during clinical supervision and in the larger organizations in which they work. However, these concerns go beyond the scope of this workbook. For helpful discussions of these topics, see *Ethics for Addiction Professionals* by LeClair Bissell and James E. Royce, *Critical Incidents: Ethical Issues in Substance Abuse Prevention and Treatment* by William White, *At Personal Risk: Boundary Violations in Professional-Client Relationships* by Marilyn Peterson, and *Sexual Dilemmas for the Helping Professional* by Jerry Edelwich and Archie Brodsky.

We want your ideas about how to improve this workbook. Please fill out the request for comments and suggestions (appendix 5) and send it to us at the address listed. Your response will help shape the content of future workbooks on this topic.

About the author. Sheila McGuire is a Licensed Social Worker and a Certified Chemical Dependency Professional. As a social worker and chemical dependency counselor, McGuire was confronted with ethical dilemmas that her training had not prepared her for. In seeking guidance from colleagues and supervisors she found that they, too, often lacked training in this area. At this time, there was little written on the topic. Fortunately, this is changing. When McGuire was asked to do a training in the area of ethics for a state hospital, it confirmed her belief that providers have a hunger to talk about professional boundaries and to teach each other. Our clients and patients benefit exponentially from the emerging dialogue on ethics—as does the helping profession as a whole.

Hazelden
Center City, Minnesota 55012-0176

Editor's note. Hazelden offers a variety of information on chemical dependency and related areas. Our publications do not necessarily represent Hazelden's programs, nor do they officially speak for any Twelve Step organization.

The personal stories in this workbook are composites of many individuals. Any resemblance to any one person, living or dead, is strictly coincidental.

Contents

Acknowledgments

This workbook is inspired by all the people who have attended training in ethics and professional boundaries. I have deep respect for all of us in the helping fields: even when we are overloaded, we will still take the risk to grapple with the complexities necessary to keep clients' needs first. We need to give ourselves a break and realize all of us have ethical dilemmas and we don't have to figure them out alone; we can help each other. The nonjudgmental teaching and mentoring we have provided each other has helped me help clients.

I am so grateful for the ethical guidance and education I have received from those who have attended my trainings and those who have presented and written on this area. I thank William White, LeClair Bissell, Marilyn Peterson, James Royce, Gary Micci, and Charlotte Chapman for reviewing all or parts of this ethics program. I thank Barb Perrin for being my first supervisor to include education on professional boundaries as a part of her supervision responsibilities.

A Challenge on Using This Workbook

As you go through this workbook, you can choose to answer many of the questions from the solid ground of theory and intellect ("Of course I know that!" "Oh, I'd never do that!" and similar variations). It is easy to know the right thing to do—out of context. My experience has shown me that clinicians with twenty years experience can still find shifting sands in the area of ethics that demands scrutiny. I hope that you reach for the emotional context in which you experience a boundary dilemma and respond from this place of growth.

Introduction: Getting the Most from This Workbook

Ethical Decision Making for Helping Professionals offers you and your staff a chance to explore how you set and maintain professional boundaries. Many discussions focus on how professionals in the helping fields cross sexual boundaries, such as dating current or former clients. With this workbook, you'll look at the more subtle boundary transgressions that can occur in any service program—and that also hurt clients. Without appropriate interventions, many of the boundaries explored in this workbook can also lead to sexual transgressions.

Our hope is that this workbook will

- Help you grasp an abstract issue such as ethics and relate it to tangible examples.
- Offer a practical framework for reflecting on ethical issues.
- Raise more questions than answers and prompt you to grapple with ethical issues.
- Offer exercises and scenarios for continuing discussion, as ethical issues continually arise in the helping fields.
- Help you think through ethical dilemmas *before* they occur, so that you can be proactive instead of reactive.

WORK WITH OTHERS

When possible, do this workbook with other colleagues. Part of the challenge in setting appropriate boundaries is seeing how our values influence our ethical decisions. Values exist on many levels—personal, cultural, and organizational. We can better clarify values when we contrast our own stance with that of other professionals. Comparing our individual choices and actions sheds new light on our sometimes unconscious motivations and values.

AVOID JUDGMENTS

Please refrain from judging yourself and others while doing this work. All of us in the helping fields have troubles with boundaries. These dilemmas just come with the territory of working with people in pain, whether physical or emotional. So be open, embrace the confusion of learning, and *be gentle*.

FOCUS ON BENEFITS

The objectives listed below describe what you can gain from *Ethical Decision Making for Helping Professionals*. By using this workbook, you can
- Create a working definition of professional boundaries (chapter 1).
- Understand how the power differential in helping relationships influences boundaries (chapter 2).
- Outline a process for making decisions that you can use when confronted with ethical dilemmas (chapter 3).
- Use checklists to spot boundary problems early on and determine your own clues for vulnerable boundaries (chapter 4).
- Recognize how ethical dictates concerning collegial relationships affect client care. Explore how dual relationships can affect our teamwork and ultimately our work with clients (chapter 5).
- Introduce self-care as a foundation for setting boundaries (epilogue).

ABOUT THE ICONS

The exercise icon signals a place for you to write, do a role play, or take other action. This workbook is not meant to be read so much as *done*. Doing the exercises will bring the topic of ethics to the level of your everyday experience.

This workbook has been designed to accompany a video entitled *Ethical Decision Making for Helping Professionals*. Indicated in the workbook text are directions for when to watch the video. If you are not using the video with this workbook, then just skip these references to the video or go to an alternate exercise as explained in the text.

A NOTE ON TERMINOLOGY

This workbook uses the words *professional* and *provider* interchangeably. Either term can include social workers, chemical dependency (substance abuse) counselors, mental health practitioners, nurses, psychologists, psychiatrists, and members of the clergy.

1. Defining Professional Boundaries

Objective: Create a working definition of professional boundaries.

A commonsense perspective on ethics is "doing the right thing because it is the right thing to do." Aristotle believed that ethics provided guidelines for virtuous action. In his rule of the *Golden Mean*, he defined the ethical choice as one that falls between two extremes. For example, trust is the virtue that lies between suspicion and foolish faith.

In our work, many ethical issues revolve around setting and maintaining professional boundaries. This, too, is a matter of balance and avoiding extremes.

Write down one possible definition of *professional boundaries*. For optimum results, work with colleagues to create this definition.

> Professional boundaries:
>
> _____
>
> _____
>
> _____
>
> _____
>
> _____

Watch the video *Ethical Decision Making for Helping Professionals* up to the STOP TAPE AND DISCUSS (1) designation. Then consider these definitions for the term *professional boundaries:*

- They are the line that separates where I end and the client begins.
- They are the emotional and physical space that gives our clients room to focus on their own healing and not on us.
- They are limits that control the professional's power so that clients aren't hurt.
- They dictate our interactions with clients.
- They're fluid limits that change depending on the client's vulnerability and our role.
- They are the parameters that keep the professional as objective as possible.

Summary: Based on your original definition and those you've just considered, in the space above, record any other definitions of professional boundaries *that will help you in your job.*

BOUNDARY TRANSGRESSIONS DEFY CATEGORIES

Sometimes we think of boundaries in terms of what areas they affect. These areas may include physical, emotional, psychological, or sexual factors. Consider the following examples.

Physical boundary transgressions
- A client comes into your office and picks up papers on your desk.
- You are meeting with a co-worker and a colleague opens the closed door, sits down, and begins talking about a crisis.
- Your supervisor hugs you without your permission after a negative performance review.

Emotional boundary transgressions
- A client shares her memories of sexual abuse with members of the support staff in a crowded waiting room.
- A staff member shares the gruesome details of her divorce during a staff meeting.
- A supervisor acts as therapist for a supervisee.

Psychological boundary transgressions
- A white client calls a black client a racist name.
- A staff member shames a co-worker by indirect criticism, ridicule, or sarcasm, such as, "Your clients sure relapse a lot. What's that say about you?"
- Your supervisor answers the phone three times during a supervisory meeting that you requested.

Sexual boundary transgressions
- A client winks at you seductively during group therapy.
- A staff member says, "Your present position—the way you're bending over—makes me think of my wild weekend. Let me tell you about it."
- A supervisor wants to know details about your clients' sex lives. Each time you try to discuss other relevant information, your supervisor steers the topic back to sex.

Although thinking in categories is useful, remember that most transgressions fit into several categories. In the examples listed above, a physical or sexual boundary merges with a psychological or emotional boundary.

BOUNDARIES ARE COMPLEX

Having a definition in hand or a clearly stated boundary can give us a false sense of security. We might assume that if we *name* the invisible line that draws a boundary, we will stop before crossing it.

For example, most helping professionals state clear limits about accepting gifts from clients. Yet, as the following exercise demonstrates, those limits can break down in daily practice.

Turn on the video starting at the STOP TAPE AND DISCUSS (1) designation and ending at the second stop and watch the scenarios about gifts. Here you will see examples of clients presenting gifts to their providers. In the space below, check (√) whether you would accept or decline the gift in each scenario.

Scenario	Accept	Decline
1.	_____	_____
2.	_____	_____
3.	_____	_____
4.	_____	_____

Summary: Now reflect on the rationale for your decisions. Write briefly about your reasons for accepting or declining any gift; then share your thoughts with your colleagues.

Note: If you are not using the video or would like to extend the exercise on gifts, then go to the exercise below.

Read each example below and check (√) whether you would accept or decline the gift. Then sum up the rationale for your decision.

1. **A client who is Hmong gives you an embroidered piece of art that depicts her personal journey in therapy.**

   ☐ Accept ☐ Decline   Rationale: _____

2. **Another client (who is not Hmong) sees the art piece from example #1 on the wall. He buys you another piece of Hmong art.**

   ☐ Accept ☐ Decline   Rationale: _____

3. **Your agency policies state that it is okay for you to accept homemade gifts from clients. A 70-year-old client gives you an ornately carved cradle. You know that she sells these cradles for $800 each.**

   ☐ Accept ☐ Decline   Rationale: _____

4. **A client gives you a greeting card. This is the third one you've received from this person in two weeks, and each time you receive the card during a group session. You sense that this client is trying to create a special relationship with you.**

   ☐ Accept ☐ Decline   Rationale: _____

Summary: Reflect on your responses to the various scenarios about accepting gifts. Discuss your ideas with colleagues. Note that one of you might accept gifts that others would not. Listen for how you and your colleagues decide which gifts are acceptable.

What guidelines will you use in the future for accepting gifts?

_____

_____

_____

What unresolved questions about accepting gifts call for more discussion?

_____

_____

_____

USING THE PROCESS

Review the steps you used in thinking about gifts from clients. You can use the same steps when discussing most boundary issues with your colleagues:

Step 1. As a group, list *specific examples* involving the boundary area in question:

> *Boundary area:* Appropriate touching
> *Example:* You hold a client's hand while she's crying during a group session.

> *Boundary area:* Self-disclosure
> *Example:* You tell a client that you take Prozac.

Step 2. Go through each example you listed in step 1 and ask, Which examples are *sometimes* okay? Which examples are *never* okay?

Step 3. Discuss individual responses. Explain the rationale for your ethical decisions.

> *This step helps us*
> - *Recognize our values.*
> - *Recognize dissonant ideas about what helps a client.*
> - *See different perspectives on what makes for an appropriate boundary.*
> - *Make explicit our process for arriving at ethical decisions.*

Step 4. Sum up any ethical decisions the group agrees on and their rationale. Outline thorny questions to address in future discussions.

CONTEXT IS KEY

As you can see, it is difficult to come up with simple guidelines for boundaries that hold true in every situation. Context—not content—often determines the appropriate boundary. In turn, context flows from many variables, including cultural norms, the type of agency, and client services offered.

Context—
not content—
often determines
the appropriate
boundary.

Say that you offer outpatient counseling. If you went to a movie with a client, you would transgress several boundaries. Yet if you were a professional in a residential setting, it may be quite appropriate for you to go to movies with clients as part of the program.

The influence of context on professional boundaries calls for us to create ethical frameworks—not simplistic answers. With constantly changing contexts, we must provide regular time to discuss boundaries in staff meetings, during clinical supervision, and with colleagues in the field.

2. The Power Differential

Objective: Understand how the power differential in helping relationships influences boundaries.

Often boundaries become clouded or get crossed because we do not remember or understand the premise behind a particular boundary. For example, why do we have boundaries concerning gifts from clients when we accept gifts from friends?

Often the answers lie in the *power differential*. This factor denies the possibility of mutual consent and calls for clear boundaries. A professional helping relationship is asymmetrical—an interaction in which the parties are not equal. We are in a position of greater authority; clients are vulnerable. We get paid; they don't. We know about their personal pain; they do not know about ours.

SCENARIO: "THE APPOINTMENT"

To get a small reminder of what it's like to be a vulnerable client, visualize the following scenario:

You are in the doctor's office. You have been sitting in the waiting room a long time; it is now 9:30, and your appointment was for 9:00. You are feeling nervous because you know something is wrong with you but you're not sure what. Perhaps you are also in pain.

You finally go up to the receptionist and ask, "How much longer will it be? My appointment was for 9:00, and I have a 10:30 meeting I have to attend."

"It won't be much longer," he answers blankly.

> Do you scream at the receptionist? No, because you are dependent on the doctor for help, and showing your true feelings might jeopardize your care. Do you say: "Forget it!" and leave? No, because you need the doctor's expertise. You can't get better on your own.

So, you sit down. Maybe you feel like crying (or screaming). Your life feels out of your control. You're behind on deadlines at work because of this illness . . . and yet you can't take care of this with your own resources, so you have to stay . . . and wait . . . and wait. Finally, your train of thought is derailed by a voice: "Excuse me, the doctor will see you now."

With relief you get up and go into the examining room, where you wait another fifteen minutes. . . . While waiting, you make a list of questions you want to ask about your illness.

The door opens and the doctor flies in with the comment, "What a crazy day! Let's see what we can do for you." She immediately begins to read your chart, making no eye contact with you.

The doctor proceeds to ask you questions, which you try to answer clearly . . . but it really is complicated, and you're confused as to when the symptoms show up or even what they are. You try to explain all this but she cuts you off. With anger rising, you find yourself thinking, Why can't I explain this? It's probably not important anyway.

You ask three of your ten questions. You don't quite understand some of the answers, and when you ask for clarification, you're still not sure if you understand but you drop it and don't ask the other questions.

The doctor gives you a possible diagnosis, although she's not sure, and prescribes some medication. She also refers you to a specialist whose office is thirty miles away.

After the appointment, while you're standing in the clinic parking lot, you realize you don't even know what the medication's side effects are. You're fuming: "Why didn't I stand up for myself! I am the one who's paying her. What's wrong with me? I don't have time to see another specialist!"

We leave the scenario here without following the wait at the drug store . . . the cost of the prescription that may or may not work . . . and the exposure you feel while sharing things about your body with a specialist you don't know.

"The appointment" scenario has been simplified in several ways. It does not reflect the following factors:
- You probably have a stronger ego than many of your clients.
- The scenario did not involve a chronic condition requiring you to see helping professionals routinely (daily, weekly, or monthly).
- Your job, family cohesion, or place of residence were not affected by the professional's involvement.
- You did not exhibit an illness with social and personal stigma attached.
- You were not in crisis.

How is "The appointment" similar to or different from what your clients experience?

_____

_____

_____

_____

Will your clients speak up directly if they don't like something you do or say? Why or why not?

_____

_____

_____

_____

Will your clients directly refuse to follow a recommendation? Why or why not?

_____

_____

_____

What creates a client's dependency on you and the associated transference?

_____

_____

_____

Does transference create safety for the clients in the healing process? If so, how?

_____

_____

_____

_____

_____

Transference takes place when your clients' needs and vulnerability shape their perception of you and the therapeutic relationship. Based on issues and relationships from the past, the client puts various "faces" on you — faces that are not your own.

Why do clients take responsibility for a professional's inappropriate behavior? As an example, review "The appointment" and consider the client's self-condemnation ("Why didn't I stand up for myself!...")

_____

_____

_____

_____

_____

_____

What assumptions might clients make about your expertise that have nothing to do with you personally?

_____

_____

_____

_____

What are sources of these expectations?

_____

_____

_____

_____

List five ways you exert power over clients on a daily basis.
Example: You choose meeting times to fit your schedule.

1. _____

2. _____

3. _____

4. _____

5. _____

How are clients vulnerable to your professional power? List specific examples.

Example: Clients have to follow through with your recommendations to meet court or county dictates.

Example: Clients have to trust your knowledge of appropriate referrals.

1. _____

2. _____

3. _____

4. _____

5. _____

Summary: After reflecting on the "The appointment," what do you want to remember when setting boundaries with clients?

Even on our worse days—when we feel unskilled and powerless— do we still have power? Return to "The appointment" for a moment. Again, put yourself in the client's place. Let's say that after you left the doctor's office, she sat down and cried because she felt totally incompetent that day. Did her professional identity still wield power over you during your appointment? If so, in what ways?

REMEMBERING THE POWER DIFFERENTIAL

When we forget about the power differential[1] or the excruciating vulnerability clients experience, boundaries get breached. We disrupt the therapeutic space that boundaries protect. We move in too close or we move too far away. Consider the following three examples.[2]

Example 1: The ideal
The professional is close enough to be emotionally involved. Clients feel protected and supported in their vulnerability. The professional is also distant enough to allow clients the autonomy they need to heal.

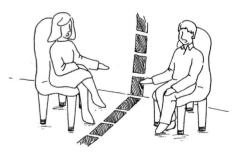

1. Discussed in depth in Marilyn Peterson's *At Personal Risk: Boundary Violations in Professional-Client Relationships,* 1993.

2. Adapted from M. Peterson's *At Personal Risk.*

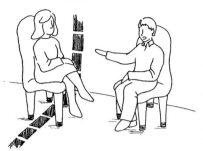

Example 2: Shrinking the boundary space

If we are uncomfortable with our power, we may reposition ourselves as buddies or peers. We come in too close. Clients may feel confused, angry, or unsafe; they know that we have more power, though we are acting as if we don't.

Example 3: Enlarging the boundary space

If we've been in too close, we might react by moving too far away. We forget clients' vulnerability and abandon them. We remove ourselves from the complex emotional relationship and thus act outside it. We may begin to think of clients as walking diagnoses—objects to be acted upon. Clients may feel alone, unheard, confused, unsafe.

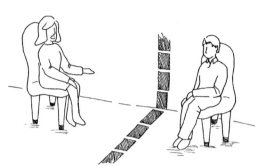

In examples 2 and 3, we reposition ourselves because we are uncomfortable with the emotional tension created by the power differential. By focusing on our own comfort, we disrupt the *integrity of care*, which directs us to always put the needs of clients first.

Read the examples below, placing yourself in the role of a provider. Note whether the professional is too close (TC), too distant (TD), or balancing distance appropriately (BD). Then discuss your answers with colleagues.

_____ **1. You think about clients as cases to get through, as charts to "finish."**

_____ **2. You talk about a client's emotional pain with colleagues while eating lunch in a full cafeteria.**

_____ **3. Your speak about your personal pain with a client.**

_____ **4. You ignore a therapeutic confrontation because you don't want the client to feel uncomfortable.**

_____ **5. You ignore a therapeutic intervention because you have an agenda you always follow at this particular time.**

_____ **6. You nod slightly when a client puts down your colleague.**

_____ **7. A client says, "I'm not ready to look at my sexual abuse." You ignore this comment and keep pushing the client for memories of abuse.**

_____ **8. You don't have time for clinical supervision this week because you're determined to finish your paperwork.**

_____ **9. You don't have time for clinical supervision this week because a client needs a special one-to-one meeting.**

____ 10. You instruct a colleague to ignore a client's complaint: "That client is always whining. She's just a manipulator. I can't stand working with her."

____ 11. You say to a client, "Your journey is just like mine. Let me tell you what helps when I'm feeling that way."

____ 12. You find yourself thinking, *Only I can help this client. This client has no one else to count on.*

____ 13. During a group session, you ignore an aside (giggling between two group members) while another client is talking.

____ 14. An entire group session consists of conversation about old cars because a charismatic client just bought a 1962 Thunderbird.

____ 15. Because a group session is going so well, you ignore the fact that it's fifteen minutes past ending time, and you decide to go for a while longer. You do this without telling your group.

____ 16. You are offering an educational component and ask the group if they mind staying an extra twenty to thirty minutes.

____ 17. As a member of a Twelve Step group, you agree to sponsor an ex-client.

____ 18. A client makes a racist slur and you ignore it.

List three of your behaviors that may signal when you are too distant from your client (underinvolved).

1. _____

2. _____

3. _____

List three *client* behaviors signaling that you may be too distant.

> **Example: An unexpected barrage of personal questions as clients try to feel closer to you.**
>
> 1. _____
>
> 2. _____
>
> 3. _____

List three of your behaviors that signal when you are too close to your client (overinvolved).

> 1. _____
>
> 2. _____
>
> 3. _____

List three *client* behaviors signaling that you may be too close.

> **Example: A seemingly unrelated burst of anger to a minor comment or request. (Clients might use anger to push you away if you have crossed their previous boundaries and are in too close.)**
>
> 1. _____
>
> 2. _____
>
> 3. _____

Because of the power differential, it is always the professional's job to set and reset boundaries with clients.

REFRAME MYTHS ABOUT BOUNDARIES

Reminder: You are only human. None of us can balance boundaries perfectly every day. If we're human, we're inconsistent. There is a myth that a competent provider *never* breaches the therapeutic space and thus *never* commits boundary transgressions. Show us such a provider and we'll show you a fictional character!

Let's reframe this myth. Competent providers are people who
- Receive routine clinical supervision and study their codes of ethics.
- Accept the complexity of maintaining boundaries.
- Admit that they have boundary dilemmas.
- Wrestle with these dilemmas and discuss them with colleagues.

3. Making Ethical Decisions

Objective: Outline a process for making decisions that you can use when confronted with ethical dilemmas.

Because maintaining boundaries in helping relationships is so complex, ethical dilemmas are guaranteed.

When you find yourself confronted with an ethical dilemma, consider how you respond:
- Do you follow a certain process to choose the most ethical action?
- Does your agency suggest a process for making ethical decisions?
- Is this process followed in staff meetings?
- Is this process followed in clinical supervision?

Below is a suggested process for making ethical decisions. Use it as a starting point as you determine what your own process will be. And whatever process you do choose, remember to keep it simple enough so that you can actually *use* it.

ONE PROCESS FOR MAKING ETHICAL DECISIONS
1. Review your code of ethics and legal mandates.
2. Seek input from a second party.
3. Determine the values (motives) involved.
4. Evaluate the long-term effects of your choices on your client.

REVIEWING YOUR LEGAL MANDATE
What are your legal mandates?
How do you find out about them
and keep updated on changes?

Note: Laws are based on specific actions in specific situations. In contrast, ethics involve contextual considerations—the various relationships involved and the ripple effects from any decision. For this reason, legal mandates can only serve as one piece in an ethical decision.

For example, many states have a legal mandate that forbids a sexual relationship between provider and client for two years after therapy terminates. But from an ethical standpoint, other questions remain. Is it okay to have a sexual relationship with an ex-client in three years? Is it ever okay to have a sexual relationship with an ex-client? Is a client ever an ex-client, and how do you decide?

REVIEWING YOUR CODE OF ETHICS

When was the last time you reviewed your code of ethics? Have a copy close at hand that you can pull out whenever you face an ethical dilemma.

Codes are minimal dictates. In helping relationships, codes serve as guidelines for reducing harm to clients that can result from the power differential. (See chapter 2 for more on the power differential.) Our ethics codes—national, state, and agency—protect the integrity of care: clients' needs come first. In her book *At Personal Risk: Boundary Violations in Professional-Client Relationships*, Marilyn Peterson states it well: "Codes are covenants that say we will give and not take."

As noted below, various codes of ethics dictate similar conduct across the helping professions.[3]

Common Elements of Ethics Codes
- Avoid dual relationships that exploit clients—socially, financially, or sexually. For example, avoid acting as a client's therapist and financial advisor.
- Avoid discriminatory behaviors.
- Restrict treatment to your areas of competence. Know your limitations. Refer the client to another professional when it is in the client's best interest.
- Respect and safeguard the autonomy of clients.
- Respect the rights, views, and clinical practices of other professionals.
- Hold colleagues accountable for ethical practices.
- Continue to grow professionally.
- Consult with other professionals when circumstances dictate. When giving direct client care, get clinical supervision.
- Adhere to all state and federal laws that govern client care, such as laws that relate to confidentiality.

Use these dictates and the suggested process for making ethical decisions as you examine the following scenarios.

At this point, you can watch the video starting at the STOP TAPE AND DISCUSS (2) designation. View the rest of the video, stopping at appropriate times to discuss the scenarios and answer the discussion questions included with the video. If you are not using the video—or if you want further issues to discuss— then proceed to the three scenarios that follow.

Note: These scenarios may not fit your work situation exactly. Please generalize. Focus on the ethical issues that would arise for you if you were in the situation described in each scenario.

---

3. The codes reviewed are those for various professional organizations, including Chemical Dependency Counselors (NAADAC), Social Workers (NASW), Psychologists (APA), Clergy (Academy of Parish Clergy), and Nurses (ANA).

SCENARIO 1: "CAN YOU GIVE ME A RIDE HOME?"

After the other group members have left, Mandy (a client) asks Bert (the provider) for a ride home. "There was a message that my usual ride can't make it," says Mandy. "I know you live near me because our phone numbers have the same first three digits."

Bert is uncomfortable with this last comment but ignores it. "Well sure, I guess, but only this one time," he says. "My supervisor, Bren, is very clear that we don't give clients rides home." As they walk to the parking lot, Rita, Bert's colleague, notices Bert getting into his car with a client.

During the ride home, Bert remembers he needs to stop at the pharmacy. "Oh, are you sick?" asks Mandy.

"No, my baby girl has an ear infection and I'll be up all night if I don't get this stuff," Bert replies. "I haven't had a full night's sleep in a week." Bert and Mandy continue to chat about Bert's baby. "Do you want to have kids?" Bert asks.

"I don't know," Mandy replies. "I had an abortion, and I've never really recovered from it. How could I have a baby after I killed my first one? Oh, here's the pharmacy."

While Bert is picking up the prescription, Mandy notices a book in the backseat titled Miscarriage and Loss. *"Oh man, he's been through a recent miscarriage, and I go and bring up my abortion!" Mandy groans. "What's wrong with me?" Mandy then digs in her purse, pulls out a five-dollar bill, and attaches a note to it that reads, "Thanks for the ride—and everything." She signs the note and puts it in the glove box.*

During group the following week, neither Mandy nor Bert bring up the ride home. Mandy feels distanced from the group because of their "secret." Parts of her special relationship with Bert (as Mandy sees it) feel great, and she thinks that Bert likes her better than the other group members. But Mandy also feels distanced from the rest of the group because of the "secret" she shares with Bert. Between guessing what she can and can't say—and worrying about Bert's pain and her own position in group—Mandy misses most of the group interaction.

At one point, Bert tries to involve Mandy. She is not sure what to disclose and feels angry at the double bind Bert has put her in. Mandy feels she'll lose no matter what she says.

Bert feels Mandy's distance from the group and is confused by these new walls. Suddenly he feels their therapy is stuck. He finds himself staying highly aware of her nonverbal cues. The next day, Bert discovers the five dollars in the glove box.

 Apply the four-step process for making ethical decisions to scenario 1.

---

1. *Review your code of ethics and legal mandates.*
   In light of your ethical codes, what boundary transgressions could be taking place in this scenario?

   _____

   _____

   _____

   What other ethical issues are raised in this scenario?

   _____

   _____

   _____

   _____

---

2. **Seek input from a second party.**
   If you were Bert, who would you talk to about the ethical issues raised in this scenario?

   _____

   _____

3. **Determine the values (motives) involved.**
   Any time we make a decision, our values come into play. It is important to make these values (motives) conscious and determine whether to
   • Keep them as they are.
   • Decide if our values impede the client's autonomy.
   • Revise our values if they undermine our present therapeutic work or fail to support the codes we've vowed to follow.

   What may be some of Bert's personal values (motives) in this scenario?

   _____

   _____

   _____

   What are possible agency values (motives) related to this scenario?

   _____

   _____

   _____

4. **Evaluate the long-term effects of your choices on your client.**
   What actions could Bert take to resolve the ethical issues raised by this scenario?

   Choice 1:

   _____

   _____

   Effects of choice 1: (Remember to consider short-term consequences as you weigh the long-term effects.)

   _____

   _____

   _____

   Choice 2:

   _____

   _____

Effects of choice 2:

_____

_____

_____

Choice 3:

_____

_____

_____

Effects of choice 3:

_____

_____

_____

What choice do you think is the most ethical?

_____

_____

_____

Discuss this scenario and your choice with colleagues. For more ideas on issues related to this scenario, see appendix 2 on page 55.

SCENARIO 2:
"SECRETS THAT KEEP US STUCK"

While reading this scenario, put yourself in the role of the provider.

Tamara is a client in your program and Martha is her primary provider. Martha and you facilitate a group together.

Before work one day, Martha flops down in your office and says, "I feel so shaky today. I just had a terrible fight with my mother." You do not have time to respond because it is time for group.

At the beginning of group, you ask for the homework assignment on "secrets that keep us stuck." Tamara crosses her arms over her chest and says, "I didn't do it. The questions don't apply to me and I've just been too busy."

Martha sighs and responds. "Tamara, this is your third homework assignment that's late. All the other members have it done. You're going to have to talk about this big secret in your life if you want to stay sober."

Tamara's face begins to turn red. "I'm just not ready to talk about it yet," she says. Martha continues to probe until you interrupt and suggest that the group move on. You do not talk with Martha after group.

After that group session, Tamara starts dropping by your office regularly. You enjoy her visits; she reminds you of your own struggles during recovery. Tamara begins to talk about her sexual abuse. You counsel her and yet suggest that she bring those issues up in group and to Martha, her primary provider.

"I don't trust Martha and I've been betrayed by groups in the past," Tamara replies. "I'm really glad I can trust you." Tamara tells you she is lesbian and is afraid that the group will find out. During the next group session, you are aware that you feel protective of Tamara.

One afternoon Martha comes by and says, "I'm concerned about Tamara. She isn't bonding with the group or looking at her sexual abuse. I think that she uses her sexuality to keep from dealing with the group."

 Apply the four-step process for making ethical decisions to scenario 2.

1. Review your code of ethics and legal mandates.
In light of your ethical codes, what boundary transgressions could be taking place in this scenario?

_____

_____

_____

What other ethical issues are raised in this scenario?

_____

_____

_____

2. Seek input from a second party.
Who would you talk to about the ethical issues involved in this scenario?

_____

_____

3. Determine the values (motives) involved.
How are your personal values (motives) involved?

_____

_____

How are your agency's values (motives) involved?

_____

_____

_____

4. *Evaluate the long-term effects of your choices on your client.*

Choice 1:

_____
_____
_____

Effects of choice 1:

_____
_____
_____

Choice 2:

_____
_____
_____

Effects of choice 2:

_____
_____
_____

Choice 3:

_____
_____
_____

Effects of choice 3:

_____
_____
_____

What choice do you think is the most ethical?

_____
_____
_____

Discuss this scenario and your choice with colleagues. For more ideas on issues related to this scenario, see appendix 2 on page 55.

SCENARIO 3: "WHAT'S UP WITH JOSH?"

This scenario raises a question: who is our client—the individual or the public?
While reading this scenario, put yourself in the role of the provider.

Josh, a client, has missed all his appointments during the last week. He has a dual diagnosis: bipolar disorder and substance abuse. You have been his primary provider. "Does anybody know what's up with Josh?" you ask during a group session. "I Don't know," another client responds, "but I saw him in Gilligan's bar last night and he was as drunk as a skunk."

Josh was referred by the courts after one incident of child molestation. This sexual offense occurred at a school playground near his home when Josh was drunk. He received treatment for alcohol abuse and followed through on all continuing care requirements for the first six months after treatment. When his continuing care group ended, Josh was referred to you for ongoing one-to-one counseling. His probation ended two weeks ago.

During counseling, one thing has become apparent: Josh perceives that his sexual offense occurred only because he was on a drinking binge. When he was on this binge, he also stopped taking his medication. Josh sees it this way: "The only time I'm dangerous and can't control my behavior is when I'm drunk. As long as I don't drink, I won't ever hurt anybody again."

You are afraid Josh will go back to the playground and perpetrate again. What will you do?

 Apply the four-step process for making decisions to scenario 3.

> **1. *Review your code of ethics and legal mandates.***
> **What ethical dictates are relevant to this scenario?**
>
> _____
>
> _____
>
> _____
>
> **It's important to stay aware of legal mandates and their ramifications. Are any legal mandates relevant to this scenario? If so, what are they?**
>
> _____
>
> _____
>
> _____
>
> **Note: It is likely that you will consider the Tarasoff case in discussing this scenario.[4] The "Duty to Warn" mandate resulted from this case. Yet there is no specific victim in this scenario or "specific means" stated by your client.**
>
> **How do you find out about legal mandates?**
>
> _____
>
> _____
>
> _____

4. *Tarasoff v. Regents of the University of California*, 131 Cal Reptr 14 (1976).

2. Seek input from a second party.
Who will you talk to about the ethical issues raised in this scenario?

_____

_____

Are these people available to you on a routine basis?

_____

When making an ethical decision, do you consult colleagues whose values differ from your own? How do you ensure that this consultation will take place?

_____

_____

Note: In his work with professionals who became sexually involved with clients, Kenneth Pope found that these professionals were usually working in isolation and always making decisions in isolation.[5] Talk to somebody!

If you lack appropriate clinical supervision, what will you do to resolve the ethical issues raised in this scenario?

_____

_____

_____

Do you ever call your ethics board to discuss a case? Consider writing this board's phone number on a copy of your ethics code for easy contact. Remember that you can call anonymously. Also see Appendix Four, which lists phone numbers for national organizations concerned with ethics in the helping professions. Call and ask to talk with someone on the ethics board or committee.

3. Determine the values (motives) involved.
How are your personal values (motives) involved?

_____

_____

_____

How are your agency's values (motives) involved?

_____

_____

_____

5.   K. S. Pope and J. C. Bouhoutsos, *Sexual Intimacy Between Therapists and Patients,* (New York: Praeger, 1986).

4. *Evaluate the long-term effects of your choices on your client.*

Choice 1:

_____

_____

_____

Effects of choice 1: (Remember to consider short-term effects as you look at long-term consequences.)

_____

Choice 2:

_____

_____

_____

Effects of choice 2:

_____

Choice 3:

_____

_____

_____

Effects of choice 3:

_____

In order to weigh long-term effects on our clients, we must know who our client is. Consider whose needs you will meet and whose interests you will serve.

How will Josh be affected by these possible choices?

_____

How will your other present clients be affected by your choices?

_____

How will future clients be affected by your choices?

_____

How will your organization be affected by your choice? (It is critical that we have documented supervision supporting an agency's stance on an ethical issue.)

_____

_____

_____

We are responsible to our community as well. Community support is essential as we address the needs our clients have for jobs, housing, and education. How will the community be affected by your choice?

_____

_____

_____

How will the helping professions as a whole be affected by your choice?

_____

_____

What choice do you think is the most ethical?
As you answer this question, think back to your code of ethics. How are these dictates supported or compromised by your choice?

_____

_____

Discuss this scenario and your choice with colleagues. For more ideas on issues related to this scenario, see appendix 2 on page 55.

BACK TO BASICS

After applying the process for making ethical decisions suggested in this chapter, you might feel overwhelmed. When we scrutinize the process, it may seem that, as one therapist put it, "any ethical decision could take forty hours and five committees to solve!"

Our intent is not to overwhelm you. Rather, the aim is for you to discover how you make decisions on a daily basis when faced with ethical dilemmas. Also remember that the four-step process suggested in this chapter is only one option. As you grapple with ethical choices, you may arrive at a process you like more.

To get back to the basics of ethical decision making, evaluate your choices with a couple of foolproof questions. For example:

- How would your mentor or role model regard your decision?
- If an article on your decision was printed in the local paper, would you still make this choice?
- Does your decision harm anyone? (For a detailed discussion of this question, see *Critical Incidents: Ethical Issues in Substance Abuse Prevention and Treatment* by William White.)

Based on your experience with the previous exercises, what is *your* preferred process for making ethical decisions?

1. _____

2. _____

3. _____

4. _____

4. Taking Inventory: When Personal Boundaries Become Vulnerable

Objective: Use checklists to spot boundary problems early on and determine your own clues for vulnerable boundaries.

Another important way to maintain professional boundaries is to take an inventory of our boundary vulnerabilities on a regular basis. We never outgrow this need.

KEEPING THE PAST IN THE PAST

Consider how your personal past affects the way you set boundaries in the present:

Provider: *You really have to forgive your mom. She's alcoholic. She didn't mean to hurt you.*

Client: *That's easy for you to say. You don't know what it's like! And it feels great to feel mad. I was always the good kid and never felt angry. And I am mad that she wasn't there for me. I grew up all alone.*

Provider: *What I hear is sadness. And I do know. My mom was alcoholic and died before we made peace. Believe me, it's not worth living with that guilt.*

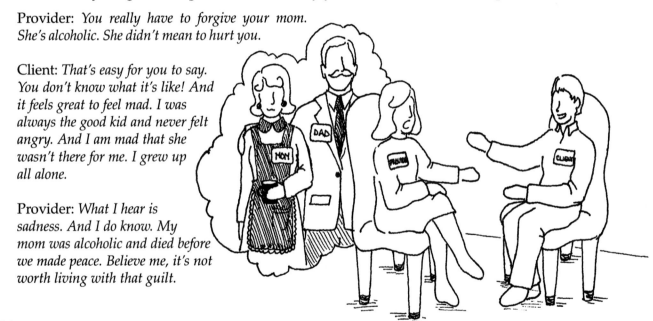

List two examples of a boundary you crossed (or might cross) due to a family history of chemical abuse, mental illness, or other illness.

1. _____

2. _____

WHAT'S IN MY SUITCASE?

Your family of origin had its own boundary rules and problems. These factors influence your present perspective. As you take inventory, a relevant question to ask is *What's in my suitcase?* That is, what personal "baggage" do you carry and how might it influence your current ethical choices?

A provider answers:

When someone uses sarcasm, I'm likely to cross boundaries. Sarcasm was used in my house as the main weapon. I really understood the damage when I learned that sarcasm comes from the Greek word meaning "to tear flesh." That sure explains the damage of psychological boundary transgressions doesn't it? Now, when a client is sarcastic, I have to be very careful of my boundaries, or else I might

- *Smother the client with my self-righteous anger and think it is my mission to change this hurtful behavior.*
- *Really distance myself from the client to protect myself.*

Both responses reflect the coping behaviors I used in growing up.

A social worker answers:

My boundary problem is triangles! When I was a kid, I was expected to be the message carrier between my three siblings and my parents. It was my job to address my sisters' hurts and grievances. I spent a lot of time trying to get my parents to change and respond. Because of this role, I have to be careful at work. It's so easy for me to create triangles between angry or hurt staff members and their supervisor. With me in the middle as message carrier and problem solver, I can get so caught up that I'm late for client appointments.

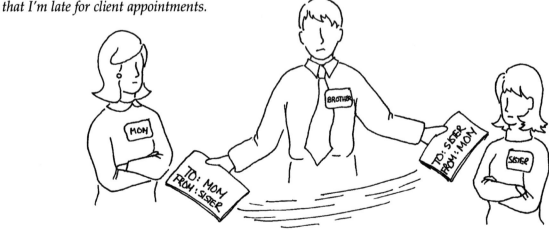

> **What were any boundary problems in your family of origin?**
>
> _____
>
> _____
>
> _____
>
> **How do these past problems play out in your present work?**
>
> _____
>
> _____
>
> _____
>
> **Because of your past, what boundaries do you need to be vigilant about?**
>
> _____
>
> _____
>
> _____

SPOTTING WINDOWS OF VULNERABILITY

Past experiences are not the only factors at work. Even in the present, personal situations outside of work can cause "windows of vulnerability" for boundaries that are usually clear:

I had just ended a twelve-year relationship and was shocked at how much self doubt and shame was flooding my grief. I had a particularly hard group. I kept trying to rescue myself from the small boundaries I was blowing. I didn't want anyone to know how incompetent I felt. The final straw was when my parents came to visit for a week to give me "support."

I finally heard the internal sirens for what they were. I went to my clinical supervision and told everyone that I was much more focused on my needs (and hiding them) than on my clients' needs. I talked about the boundary problems I thought I was having, and they actually pointed out a few more. It felt terrible, and yet they helped me monitor my behavior and client focus.

I learned so much and it was such a relief not to have to do this alone. Plus I knew clients were protected. Now I'm particularly careful of my boundaries at work when I've experienced personal rejection.

Consider situations in your present life that can cause boundary problems for you at work. Describe three specific ways your boundaries at work have been affected by external, personal issues.

1. _____

2. _____

3. _____

How do you fortify your boundaries when these things happen?

_____

_____

What situations at your work could create windows of vulnerability for boundaries that are usually clear? Give an example.

_____

_____

_____

_____

_____

_____

_____

_____

_____

_____

_____

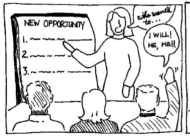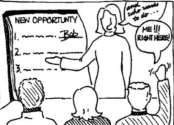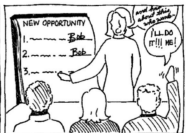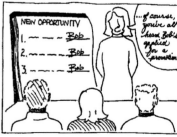

COUNTER-TRANSFERENCE:
DISCOVERING CLIENTS WHO "HOOK" YOU

Our responses to certain clients can also give us clues to possible boundary vulnerabilities. Think of a client who "hooks" you. You're *hooked* when you have strong emotional responses to a particular client. You might even describe yourself as being hypersensitive to this person.

Hypersensitive responses fall into two broad categories:

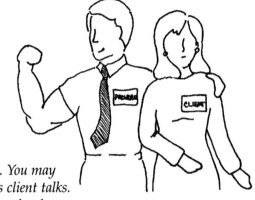

> **Seduction:** *Seduction occurs when you* really *want a client to like you and approve of you. What's more, your desire for this client to succeed is especially strong when compared to other clients. Seduction causes such actions as special favors, bending the rules, and working harder than the client.*

> **Aversion:** *Aversion takes place when a client really bugs you. You may find that your jaw clenches or your stomach churns when this client talks. Aversion causes such actions as coming down harder, more quickly, or with more severe consequences when working with one client—even when other clients do the same things. When feeling aversion, you may also ignore boundary transgressions by a client because you feel anger or even rage. You decide to wait it out and calm down. But when you do calm down, you just want to avoid the whole incident. You might feel relieved when this client switches to another agency or doesn't show for an appointment.*

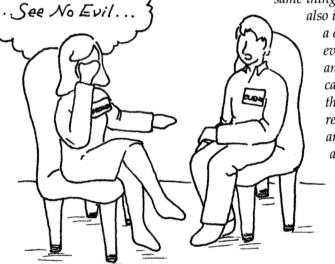

Whether you are feeling seduction or aversion, you're aware of one client's verbal and nonverbal responses much more than other clients' responses.

Think of a client who "hooks" you in a seductive way. What client characteristics and behaviors are involved?

_____

_____

What boundary problems could result from this seduction?

_____

_____

Why does this type of client seduce you, and what does your answer tell you about yourself?

_____

_____

Now think of a client toward whom you feel aversion. What client characteristics and behaviors "hooked" you in this way?

_____

_____

What boundary problems could result from this aversion?

_____

_____

Why do you feel aversion to this type of client, and what does your answer tell you about yourself?

_____

_____

CLUES TO POSSIBLE BOUNDARY PROBLEMS

If boundaries are so fluid, then how do you know when there is a boundary concern? One answer is to create checklists of your own thoughts, feelings, and behaviors—especially those that signal vulnerable boundaries. This checklist can tell you when it's time to pull out your process for making ethical decisions and talk to someone.

Consider the following list of thoughts and feelings. How do they relate to you? Do you see them as signals of potential boundary problems? Rate each item using this scale:
- N= Never indicates a potential boundary problem
- S = Sometimes indicates a potential boundary problem
- A= Almost always indicates a potential boundary problem

_____ 1. **I feel obsessed with a particular client or situation.**

_____ 2. **I feel hypersensitive when I'm around a particular client or group. (Strong transference or counter-transference is involved.)**

_____ 3. **I feel that I have a secret. (Note: Shame and guilt are often involved in boundary transgressions.)**

_____ 4. **I'm afraid that a client will get angry with me.**

_____ 5. **I'm afraid that a client will not like me.**

_____ 6. **I wish that a client or situation would just disappear.**

_____ 7. **I hope the client doesn't let anybody else know about what I said or did.**

_____ 8. **I feel a prolonged sense of incompetence.**

_____ 9. **I'm anxious and worried that my words and actions will make or break a client's healing.**

_____ 10. **I feel stuck, as if therapy is not progressing.**

_____ 11. **I feel like a care*taker* and not a care*giver*.**

_____ 12. **I feel panicked, pressed to do something *quickly* to take care of it—whatever "it" is.**

_____ 13. **I have sexual feelings toward a client (even if it's only in one session).**

_____ 14. **I'm in a double bind. Any way I go with this client will only make the situation worse.**

_____ 15. **I think that staff members are avoiding me.**

_____ 16. **I feel judgmental. I think that most or all of the other staff members are too rigid (or too loose) in setting boundaries with clients.**

_____ 17. **I think that no one understands my work with this client.**

_____ 18. **I enjoy client compliments that build me up by putting another provider down. For example: "You're the *best* counselor in this place, not like Marty."**

_____ 19. **I feel angry at clients for their "slow progress." I take the client's progress personally.**

_____ 20. **I resent a co-worker who brings up a concern about boundaries.**

_____ 21. **I believe a client's compliment is purely about me and does not involve transference.**

_____ 22. **I feel obligated to meet a client's demands although they go beyond what I provide to other clients.**

Summary: Review the items in the list above. Then add any other thoughts or feelings that signal a possible boundary problem for you.

Consider the following list of behaviors. How do they relate to you? Do you see them as signals of potential boundary problems? Rate each item using this scale: N = Never indicates a potential boundary problem
S = Sometimes indicates a potential boundary problem
A = Almost always indicates a potential boundary problem

_____ 1. **I avoid a particular client or situation.**

_____ 2. **I find myself working harder than a client.**

_____ 3. **I'm lax about following through on my commitments at work.**

_____ 4. **I act in ways that undermine organizational rules, expectations, and values.**

_____ 5. **I scrutinize my clothing on the days when I meet with a certain client.**

_____ 6. **I avoid clinical supervision. Or I attend but avoid discussing "that particular case."**

_____ 7. **I reverse roles, such as asking the client to be in charge or seeking emotional understanding from the client.**

_____ 8. **I give clients gifts or accept gifts that go beyond acceptable policy limits.**

_____ 9. **I hold one client accountable in a unique way, even when this is not part of the treatment plan. (This includes special treatment in any form.)**

_____ 10. **I take a client's feelings "home" with me.**

_____ 11. **I practice extended self-sharing with a client.**

_____ 12. **I talk more during a session than the client does.**

_____ 13. **I get more personal satisfaction from my work than from my life outside of work.**

_____ 14. **I continue the helping relationship with clients outside my unit or agency walls, even when doing so is not part of my job.**

_____ 15. **I seek personal friendships or sexual relationships with clients or ex-clients.**

_____ 16. **I stop attending conferences and seminars that challenge my methods of treatment.**

Summary: Review the items listed in the previous exercise. Then list any other behaviors that signal a possible boundary problem for you.

BOUNDARIES ENTER TREATMENT WITH OUR CLIENTS

When it comes to setting boundaries, clients have their own strengths and weaknesses. It is important to respect and respond to the boundary history and vulnerabilities of each client. Remember that clients bring their own suitcases full of boundary history with them.

Boundary histories are different for each client just as they are different for each provider. Consider this example:

Lorene (a client) asks where you grew up. When you answer, she says, "Hey, I grew up in Kitop too! That's great! Do you remember the Korn

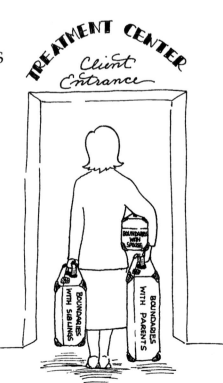

Festival?" For Lorene, your disclosure helped to create trust and deepened the therapeutic relationship. Because of your shared background, she believes you can understand her better.

Her belief reflects her personal history. Lorene's family of origin treated self-disclosure with kindness and respect. They kept private information private.

Thomas (another client) also asks where you grew up. When you answer, he says, "I grew up in Kitop, too. Oh, wow . . . I suppose you went to the Korn Festival." For Thomas, your disclosure creates a rift in the therapeutic relationship. He feels unsafe because he fears you might tell someone back home about his treatment. Or, you might know something about him that he doesn't want you to know.

Given his personal history, this is not surprising. In Thomas's family of origin, nothing was private. His father gathered information by listening in on phone conversations and going through Thomas's drawers. He would then use the information to ridicule Thomas.

Remember that clients uphold or challenge boundaries
- To keep important people responding to them (whether positively or negatively) the way they did when growing up.
- To adjust or establish a therapeutic distance that currently feels most safe to them.
- To test and ensure that the boundaries they need to do their own healing are indeed in place. For example, clients who survive incest may test providers by approaching them sexually.
- To develop autonomy. For example, adolescents may test limits as part of their growth and development.
- To mirror what they see as normal behavior, influenced by the above factors plus peer norms and social norms.

> *Think about how many movies portray professionals dating, being sexual with, or befriending their clients or members of clients' families. To begin, consider* The Prince of Tides *or* The Color of Night. *Also note how many television sitcoms use boundary breaches as a basis for humor.*

It is essential that we assess what needs the client is actually trying to meet through a boundary challenge. Then we can meet the need while still setting limits. Though a client's initial reaction to a limit may be, for example, frustration and rejection, in the long term the client will feel safe and relieved.

Think about boundary challenges that your clients initiate. Working with colleagues, brainstorm a list of examples.

When we set boundaries with clients, it helps to understand and internalize the therapeutic premise for the boundary.

Consider what happens when you forget to internalize the premise for a boundary. You're more likely to set a boundary with a rationale such as "That's just the rule" or "My supervisor says so." (For an example, see the scenario titled "Can you give me a ride home?" on page 19.)

Setting boundaries in such an indirect way can give a false impression: If it weren't for this rule, I'd go ahead and do it. When you set a limit indirectly, clients may get confused. Most likely they'll try to challenge another boundary to figure out where you stand. Remember, though the client may initiate the boundary transgression, it is always *the provider's responsibility to uphold and reset the appropriate boundary.*

Some ways that clients challenge boundaries:

- *Asking for your home phone number.*
- *Flirting with you.*
- *Asking for special favors.*
- *Talking negatively about another staff member.*
- *Asking for personal information about another staff member.*
- *Reading papers on your desk.*
- *Routinely arriving early for an appointment just to chat.*
- *Routinely asking for advice ("Just tell me what to do").*

From the previous exercise, choose one boundary challenge that your clients initiate and list it here:

_____

_____

What is the therapeutic premise for the boundary involved here? In other words, how does the boundary promote client care? Write down the actual words you'd use to explain this premise to the client or a colleague.

_____

_____

What is the client trying to tell you through this boundary challenge? What needs might the client be trying to meet?

_____

_____

How will you assess and address this need in your response to the boundary challenge? Again, write down the actual words you'd use in speaking to the client.

_____

_____

This exercise can be done as a role play involving a client and provider. If no one is available to role play with you, then write out a script for a role play.

Review the earlier exercise on boundary challenges that your clients initiate (see page 39.) Choose one example you listed there. Explain the therapeutic premise for the boundary involved here, using the actual words you'd say to the client.

Provider: _____

_____

_____

_____

Now write down the response you'd expect from the client. Remember that when we first set a limit, clients will often feel angry, defensive, hurt, rejected, misunderstood, or ashamed.

Client: _____

_____

_____

_____

Next, speak or write down what you'd say to this response. Continue in this manner with several more exchanges between client and provider. Use additional paper if needed.

Provider: _____

_____

_____

_____

Client: _____

_____

_____

_____

Provider: _____

_____

_____

_____

Client: _____

_____

_____

_____

Summary: Was it hard to be explicit in explaining the premise for the boundary? If so, what specifically was hard for you?

_____

_____

_____

Were you able to understand and articulate the premise for the boundary? If not, who will you talk to?

_____

_____

Have you internalized this premise? If not, what steps will you take so you *can* internalize it?

_____

_____

What needs do you think the client was trying to meet in this exchange?

_____

_____

Discuss your responses with colleagues.

RESPECTING CLIENTS' BOUNDARIES

In any case, *if we teach clients to respect boundaries, we need to respect the boundaries they set.* This means accepting our clients' autonomy and their need for limits that are different from our own. Labeling a client as "resistant" can be one way to disregard a client's preferred boundaries.

Clients set boundaries in many ways, such as refusing to share feelings or family information. Again, it is important for us to understand the therapeutic need for the boundary and respond accordingly. *It's always the job of the provider to monitor the boundary.* We may need to revisit the situation and reset the boundary once we understand the problem—even if this takes weeks.

SETTING BOUNDARIES EXPLICITLY

Consider the benefits and drawbacks of explicitly stating the premise for a boundary. Doing so with a client may

- Help *us* understand the premise—even if the client doesn't.
- Help us to internalize and thus uphold the boundary.
- Keep our behavior aligned with the boundary.
- Provide a role model for setting limits.
- Teach the client what to expect from other providers. (Do you have an educational piece about boundaries for your clients?)
- Help clients who've had previous education on therapeutic boundaries.

Some drawbacks of stating the premise may be that

- It makes more sense to just *act* on the premise because of time limitations or context.
- Explanations allow us to manipulate a client's response. For example, we might state a premise because we don't want the client to be mad at us.

Working with colleagues, create your own list of the benefits and drawbacks of explicitly setting boundaries with clients.

Benefits: _____

_____

_____

_____

Drawbacks: _____

_____

_____

_____

Summary: Take a minute to write down two boundaries you need to set or reset with clients to ensure the integrity of care—that the client's needs come first.

1. _____

2. _____

---

5. Boundaries between Colleagues

Objectives: Recognize how ethical dictates concerning collegial relationships affect client care. Explore how dual relationships can affect our teamwork and ultimately our work with clients.

FOCUSING ON CLIENT CARE

In order to keep a system focused on client care, we need to monitor and maintain our boundaries with co-workers. For example, when you're angry with a colleague or distrust a co-worker, where is your energy going? The amount of energy we expend in self-protection, anger, and indirect fighting with co-workers takes away from what we can give to our clients—immediately and in the long term.

If we don't quickly clean up boundary problems with co-workers, we can increase our burnout potential. In the long term, we may have less and less to give our clients. Ideally, our co-workers should be a source of replenishment, not a source of depletion. Besides, who wants to work in a place that is any more stressful than it has to be? We spend a good portion of our lives at work, and most of us want to have fun there.

That's why our ethic codes dictate that we
Respect the rights, views, and clinical practices of other professionals.

While at the same time these codes direct us to
Hold colleagues accountable for ethical practices.

This works both ways—we also will be held accountable—which leads to another ethical dictate:
Continue to grow professionally.

How are these three dictates related? And how often do we manipulate the first dictate to avoid the other two? Keep these questions in mind as you read the next scenario.

SCENARIO: "HAVE YOU TALKED TO HIM?"

You walk into your clinical supervision group with relief. You have a pressing concern about a client you are meeting with tomorrow.

Your clinical supervisor asks who wants to go first. Before you can breathe, John, a co-worker, jumps in and starts. Your jaw clenches immediately. You cross your arms and begin thinking, He always goes first. Now none of us will get any time. He just talks and talks. I think he creates dependency in his clients. They all worship the ground he walks on and don't feel that they can do anything without his guidance. That's really disrespectful.

Your consciousness returns to group, and you realize you have missed most of John's case setup. It doesn't matter. He doesn't listen to supervision anyway, *you say to yourself.*

By now you are furious at John and at the group for not holding John accountable. After John has gone on and on and on (in your opinion), it's time for another case. At this point you feel too distracted and angry to talk about your case. Supervision ends without you getting the clinical help you need.

As you walk back to your office with Luis, a co-worker, you grumble, "I can't stand that John. He puts his ego needs before his clients. I hate being in group with him."

"Have you talked to him?" Luis asks.

"Are you kidding?" you say. "Besides, he has a right to work differently than I do."

In what ways are you respecting John's rights, views, and ethical practices?

_____

_____

In what ways are you *not* showing that respect?

_____

_____

Do you *feel* respectful toward John?

How does your response affect the integrity of service—to put client care first?

_____

_____

How is the dictate "hold colleagues accountable for ethical practices" affected by your response?

_____

_____

How is the dictate to "continue to grow professionally" affected?

_____

_____

Summary: Can we respect colleagues if we do not hold them accountable for what we view as ethical breaches? Explain your answer.

_____

_____

Respect means forming an opinion only after hearing your colleague's point of view. How do we fail to follow this guideline, and what are the consequences?

_____

_____

How do you want your colleagues to help you grow professionally?

_____

_____

Whenever you have conflicts with co-workers, consider taking a mini-inventory. Think of one staff member who is driving you "nuts" right now.

Is your jaw clenching or your stomach churning? Good. Now answer the questions below:

What boundaries am I not upholding in my response to this colleague?

_____

_____

With myself? _____

_____

With my colleague? _____

_____

What boundaries do I need to (re)establish so I can serve clients better?

_____

_____

With myself? _____

_____

With my colleague? _____

_____

DUAL RELATIONSHIPS AMONG CO-WORKERS

There are many kinds of relationships going on at any worksite. Overlapping roles with co-workers make boundary setting even harder. It is difficult and scary to approach a co-worker with a boundary concern. This action becomes even more difficult when layers of relationships exist among the staff.

Author David Powell offers a useful definition to consider: "A dual relationship exists when one person interacts with another in more than one capacity at the same time, so as to suggest the possibility of an ethical compromise or conflict of interest."[6]

Dual relationships among staff members can be great—and they can be a nightmare. We gain by making dual relationships explicit. Then we can decide if such relationships energize or deplete the staff by positively or negatively affecting the team, and thus clients.

Even when a dual relationship with a co-worker is positive for you, it might affect other staff members in ways that are unexpected.

Say that you and a co-worker play in the same softball league after work. You've also set very clear boundaries with this person. For example, you *never* talk about work outside of work. Answer these questions:

> **How would this relationship be perceived by the rest of the staff?**
>
> _____
>
> _____
>
> **Would your colleagues *know* about the boundary you've set? Will they trust that the boundary is upheld?**
>
> _____
>
> _____
>
> **Even if the dual relationship is explicit, would colleagues feel that the relationship is affecting work? Can colleagues raise their concerns?**
>
> _____
>
> _____

6. David J. Powell with Archie Brodsky, *Clinical Supervision in Alcohol and Drug Abuse Counseling: Principles, Models, Methods* (Lexington, Mass.: Lexington Books, 1993).

Brainstorm a list of the dual relationships that can exist in any organization. For example, co-workers may play in the same bowling league, serve on the same church board, eat lunch together every day, be best friends, or date.

_____
_____
_____
_____
_____
_____
_____
_____
_____
_____
_____
_____
_____
_____
_____
_____
_____
_____
_____
_____
_____
_____
_____
_____
_____
_____
_____
_____
_____
_____
_____
_____
_____

Fill in the chart at right, listing examples of dual relationships along with their possible positive and negative effects. Four broad categories of dual relationships are included. If you are doing this exercise as a large group, divide into smaller groups. Each small group can discuss one or two categories. Then meet again as a large group to share your responses.

DUAL RELATIONSHIPS

Family relationships
Example: Co-workers have a blood relationship.

Social relationships with peers
Example: Co-workers are daily "lunch buddies."

Supervisor/supervisee relationships
Example: Co-workers were once peers and best friends; now one supervises the other.

Antagonistic relationships
Example: Co-workers are at philosophical odds.

POSITIVE EFFECTS	NEGATIVE EFFECTS
Example: They may be able to solve conflict more easily.	Example: External conflict may contaminate the worksite.
Example: They get re-energized and have more fun.	Example: They talk only about work, so lunch is not a break from work.
Example: They may be more open and honest with each other.	Example: The supervisee may not accept supervision well.
Example: With appropriate conflict resolution, colleagues can challenge and learn from each other.	Example: The conflict creates a hurricane of negativity that drains the staff's energy.

Summary: Review your responses to the exercise on pages 48–49. Which dual relationships had more negative effects than positive effects? (Consider the number of effects you identified *and* the magnitude of each effect.)

_____

_____

_____

What can you and your organization do to reduce these negative effects?

_____

_____

_____

Which dual relationships had more positive effects than negative effects? Again, consider the number of effects you listed, as well as their magnitude.

_____

_____

_____

What can you and your organization do to support these positive effects?

_____

_____

_____

What possible behaviors at your worksite tell you that a dual relationship is hurting the staff team and thus client care?

_____

_____

_____

Are these behaviors a team issue (to be discussed as a team) or an individual issue (to be discussed person-person)?

_____

_____

_____

What, if any, policies should be in place regarding dual relationships among your staff members?

_____

_____

_____

Sometimes social relationships among co-workers can have the same effects as family relationships among co-workers. If your organization has a policy against nepotism, does this policy apply to best friends? *Should* this policy apply to best friends?

_____

_____

_____

To close this chapter, write down two boundaries you need to set or reset with co-workers to insure the integrity of care; that our clients' needs come first.

1. _____

_____

_____

_____

2. _____

_____

_____

_____

Epilogue: Caring for Ourselves So We Can Care for Others

Objective: Introduce self-care as a foundation for setting boundaries.

---

*Paradox: We can't keep our clients' needs first unless we keep **our** needs first. When we take care of ourselves, we can better take care of clients.*

By upholding personal boundaries between clients, colleagues, and supervisors, we get our professional needs met so that we can focus on clients. If we do not take the time and energy to fulfill our personal needs outside of work, we *will* fulfill them—at work. By upholding boundaries, we meet personal needs so that we don't ask clients to meet them.

To consider the balance between your personal and professional lives, answer the following questions:

> **Are you working regular overtime? (Impaired providers often start out as overworkers.)**
>
> _____

Are your personal relationships "fifty-fifty"? That is, do you get as much from these relationships as you give?

_____

Do you take all of your vacation days?

_____

Do you have friends who are not related to your work?

_____

Do you have friends who are not in the helping fields?

_____

Do you play as hard as you work?

_____

Do you really "leave" work at work?

_____

Are you having fun in your life?

_____

Who are your mentors? _____

_____

_____

What characteristics of theirs do you admire? _____

_____

_____

Add other questions that can help you keep work and life separate.

_____

_____

_____

_____

_____

Appendix One: Worksheet for Making Ethical Decisions

This worksheet summarizes the four-step process for making ethical decisions explained in this workbook. For a more detailed discussion of this process and examples of its application, see chapter 3.

1. **Review your code of ethics and legal mandates.**
2. **Seek input from a second party.**
3. **Determine the values (motives) involved.**
4. **Evaluate the long-term effects of your choices on your client.**

Choice 1 and its effects: _____

_____

_____

_____

Choice 2 and its effects: _____

_____

_____

_____

Choice 3 and its effects: _____

_____

_____

_____

What choice do you think is most ethical? _____

_____

_____

_____

Appendix Two:
Taking Scenarios Further

This appendix illustrates how the scenarios in this workbook can fuel continuing discussion. Included below are additional points and questions for you to consider when making ethical decisions about the scenarios in chapter 3. Many of these considerations apply to other scenarios as well.

Scenario 1: "Can you give me a ride home?" (page 19)
Consider these dictates from ethics codes:
- Avoid dual relationships—emotional, social, or financial.
- Seek continued professional growth and clinical supervision.
- Respect and support client autonomy.
- Hold colleagues accountable for ethical practices.
- Keep client care first.

Other ethics issues to consider:
- Acting outside your defined role can lead to role ambiguity. This, in turn, can lead to boundary ambiguity.
- Creating special relationships with certain clients isolates those clients from their peers.
- Watch for role reversal: In the client's eyes, the provider becomes the person to be helped.
- When secrets exist, triangles can occur: One client feels caught between a provider and other clients.
- Double binds can occur. For example, Mandy feels she'll lose no matter how she responds.
- Providers risk inappropriate self-disclosure.
- Think about the therapeutic space we uphold with boundaries. When was Bert too close or too distant?

Scenario 2: "Secrets that keep us stuck" (page 21)
Consider these dictates from ethics codes:
- Hold colleagues accountable for ethical practices.
- Respect the rights and views of other professionals.
- Seek out consultation and receive clinical supervision.
- Do not discriminate on the basis of sexual orientation, race, ethnicity, or culture.
- Know your limitations and areas of competence.
- Support client autonomy.

- Commit to professional growth.
- Avoid dual relationships—emotional or sexual.
- Practice confidentiality.

Other ethics issues to consider:
- Respect the boundaries set by clients. We confuse clients when we tell them to set boundaries and then ignore them.
- Role reversal takes place when the provider's needs come before the client's.
- Watch for counter-transference.
- Handle secrets carefully. What facts and feelings are inappropriate for clients to share with a group?
- Watch for missed therapeutic moments. How might providers act out boundary transgressions the client has experienced in the past?
- Special treatment can isolate clients from their peers and create triangles.
- Avoidance can signal boundary problems.
- Paternalism can undermine client autonomy.
- Does this scenario create fertile ground for breaching sexual boundaries? If so, how?

Scenario 3: "What's up with Josh?" (page 24)

Consider these dictates from ethics codes:
- Seek out consultation and receive clinical supervision.
- Know legal mandates and their implications, including confidentiality and the Tarasoff case.
- Support client autonomy.
- Know your limitations and areas of competence.

Other ethics issues to consider:
- How can hearsay (what clients say about each other) be misused?
- What is our responsibility when a client disappears?
- When does a client who disappears stop being a client?
- Would you call Josh's probation officer?
- Is the client's written release still active?
- Does the community have a right to know when a client presents only a general threat to safety?
- How do we monitor the effects of social pressure and emotionally charged statements on our ethical decisions?
- Is the best therapeutic stance always void of personal values? Is it possible to be morally objective?

Appendix Three:
Case Studies for Discussion

These case studies are excerpted with permission from *Ethics for Addiction Professionals* by LeClair Bissell and James E. Royce (Center City, Minn.: Hazelden, 1994).

These are all actual cases. Details have been modified to avoid identification of individuals. Answers should be based on such questions as What rights are involved? Whose rights take priority? Why? What values are at stake?

You are a certified addiction counselor in a private practice. A client comes for assessment of her son. You see a complex mother-child conflict and warn her that the assessment may take four hours, including a test. She later complains to another professional that you have overcharged her. He agrees with her and says it should not have taken that long. How do you handle it? Did the other professional act unethically?

***

Treatment Center X offers to pay a fee directly to an intervention specialist. The interventionist refuses, saying she considers this unethical, a conflict of interest, but if the treatment center wishes to reimburse the family for up to four hundred dollars of her fee, the family would be responsible for the balance. Who is right: the interventionist or the treatment center? Why?

***

An interventionist refers an overtly suicidal alcoholic and three-time loser in standard alcoholism treatment programs to a ninety-day residential center with excellent psychiatric staff specializing in dual diagnosis cases. The alcoholism treatment center to which the interventionist usually referred patients complained that he was breaking their tacit agreement. Did the center act professionally?

***

You are the EAP counselor in a firm. An alcoholic employee whom you have been counseling—now in early sobriety—admits to you he has been embezzling large sums of money from the firm. You are a trusted employee of the firm. Must you inform them? May you? What should you do?

Appendix Four: Sources of Help for Ethics Questions

American Nurses Association
1-202-651-7000

American Psychological Association
1-202-336-5500

International Certification Reciprocity Consortium
1-919-781-9734

National Association of Alcoholism and Drug Abuse Counselors
1-800-548-0497

National Association of Social Workers
1-800-638-8799

Your local ethics board or committee
(List the phone number here.) _____

For price and order information, or a free catalog,
please call our Telephone Representatives.

HAZELDEN

1-800-328-9000
(Toll Free. U.S., Canada,
and the Virgin Islands)

1-612-257-4010
(Outside the U.S.
and Canada)

1-612-257-1331
(24-Hour FAX)

Pleasant Valley Road • P.O. Box 176 • Center City, MN 55012-0176